PREMED FOR PARENTS

What You Need to Know When your Child Says that he (or she) Wants to Be a Doctor

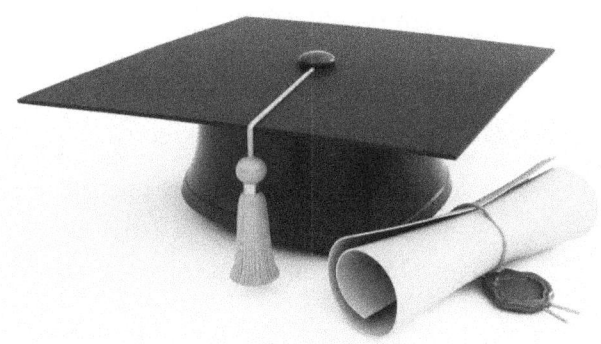

By
Ronald Kapp, MD, PhD
PreMed Advisor to the Elite College Student

Cover Design: S. Verstappen

Woodbridge Press

Toronto, Canada

PREMED FOR PARENTS

What You Need to Know When your Child Says that he
(or she) Wants to Be a Doctor

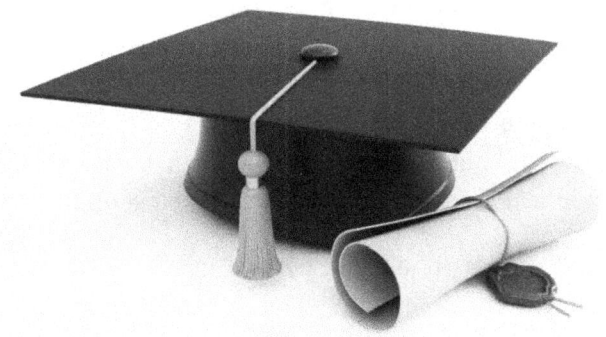

COURSE DISCLAIMER

This *PreMed For Parents* book is designed to educate and provide general information to the undergraduate premedical student. It is sold with the understanding that the publisher and author are not providing legal or professional services. Because each student is different, specific advice should be tailored to the particular circumstances. For this reason, the student is advised to consult with his or her campus premedical advisor for specific course requirements.

The author has taken reasonable precautions in the preparation of this book and believes the facts and recommendations are accurate as of the date it was written. However, neither the author nor the publisher assume any responsibility for acceptance or rejection by any medical school admissions committee. Getting accepted into medical school is not an easy challenge. It will continue to require hard work and a dedicated effort on the part of the student. The author and publisher specifically disclaim any liability resulting from the use or application of the information contained in this book.

The student should use this book as a general guide and not as the ultimate source on premedical requirements. This book is meant to educate and entertain. The publisher and author assume no liability to any person or entity for any loss, damage or harm caused by, or assumed to have been caused, directly or indirectly, by the opinions or recommendations presented in this manuscript.

TABLE OF CONTENTS

HOW TO USE THIS BOOK

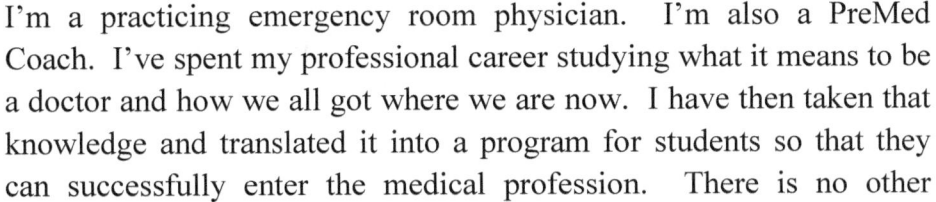

I'm a practicing emergency room physician. I'm also a PreMed Coach. I've spent my professional career studying what it means to be a doctor and how we all got where we are now. I have then taken that knowledge and translated it into a program for students so that they can successfully enter the medical profession. There is no other program like this. I can unequivocally state that no college or university campus has such a program – but more about that later.

Getting Accepted Into Medical School is competitive and emotional. Many students either give up or get rejected. However, it doesn't have to be that way and oftentimes I have seen that your parental involvement can make a huge difference. In fact, your help is often the pivotal factor between success and failure.

This book was specifically written for the parents of students that I coach. I have made it required reading for all parents and I then discuss the entire process with each parent, together and separately, so that we are all on the same wavelength, so to speak. You should understand that the material I have presented herein presupposes that your child is already one of my PreMed students and some of the assumptions and language I use may not be common knowledge outside the domain of my *Advanced PreMed Life Support* Course.

If you're interested in working with me as a Personal PreMed Coach for your son or daughter, please email me at www.kappmd.com.

My schedule is extremely tight and I only accept a few students each year. The earlier and sooner you get in touch with me, the more likely it is that I'll be able to work with you and assist your son or daughter on their path to becoming a doctor.

Even if you decide that having a Personal PreMed Coach is not to your liking, this book will still teach you a tremendous amount on how to be a "Supportive PreMed Parent." The information I present in this book will go a long way on getting your child on a successful track to gaining acceptance into medical school. Simply follow the advice in this book and I know that your child will already be ahead of 75% of premedical majors on most college campuses.

SECTION I – Simply Getting Started

Medicine is a continually evolving profession. The entire process of training to become a doctor is also always in flux. Course requirements change, new MCAT (medical college admission test) formats, different applicant pools, changing med school admissions committee members – rarely is much the same – and yet everything stays the same year after year.

This unusual paradox of it's the same as last year, only different is unique to medicine. Many parents are already doctors themselves – but I guarantee you that it's a different arena than it was 15 or 20 years ago.

SECTION I has a simple goal of getting you, the parent, in alignment with me and your son or daughter. This is a critical and fundamental requirement to success. You know the old saying, "the first step is the most important," so read and think about SECTION I material before moving on to the next Section.

SECTION II – The Foundations of Being a PreMed Parent

Many PreMed students have doctors for parents – and that is a big help. Usually, but not always. It's much different being the Parent of a Premed Student, than being the Premed student yourself. There is a different perspective, different beliefs, and even a different knowledge base. Unless you have seriously taken the time to think about what your child is trying to accomplish, you can be either a help or a hindrance.

Your child will quickly know much more than you about the mechanics of what it takes to get accepted into med school. But you are still their parent and have a big responsibility as a facilitator, a sounding board, and a behind-the-scene source of power driving your offspring to success.

I'll also provide you a quick parental summary of the action steps that you need to take to help get your child on that PreMed Path. Take a short break after reading SECTION II before moving on to the action.

SECTION III – Developing your Personal PreMed Team

PreMed should be a fun and exciting time for everyone. I'll provide you the know-how that is absolutely needed by every parent who wants the best for his or her child.

I'll show you when to intervene, when not to intervene and maybe even when to drastically change direction. I will describe to you the unique concept of why and how to develop your "personal premed team" – a concept not on any college campus today that I am aware of.

I'll also outline what steps you need to take throughout your child's career to keep him or her on track for admissions success and beyond.

Let's Get the Ball Rolling and see if Being the Parent of a Doctor is in your future.

INTRODUCTION

Dear Parent(s),

What parent doesn't want his or her child to become a doctor or a lawyer? "Here's my son, the Doctor." You think about it, you dream about it, you talk about it and you hope your child can become successful doing something like that. And then one day out of the blue you hear, *"Hey Mom, I think maybe I want to be a doctor."*

That's one common scenario. Another might go like this: You child heads off to college. You don't think much of it since it seems like everybody is "going to college these days." Every so often your child comes home on break and life seems like it really hasn't changed much. One day, late in his (or her) Senior Year of college, your child hands you that just-received acceptance letter into medical school and you are taken completely by surprise. *"What's this?"* you ask.

Here's another way it might go: Somewhere during your children's education, he (nowadays, it is just as often to be your daughter) tells you that he is "majoring in PreMed." You say great, but you really don't know what that means, what he has to do or what is going to happen. PreMed – the Great Unknown for most parents is something few know much about. In fact, most students don't know much about being an undergraduate premedical major either and they simply "learn as they go." Of course, that is a major mistake but that is a completely different subject than what is being covered in this book, PreMed for Parents.

The subject written about in this book has never been written about before. This book is for the PARENTS of undergraduate PreMed students who are trying to get accepted into medical school. It is the result of over 20 years of personal research into not just how to get accepted into medical school, but also of how to be a successful doctor after you finish medical school.

The entire process is competitive, grueling and emotional – and I mean from start to finish. Getting accepted into medical school is only the first step along a 40 year journey. It is a fact that over 50% of today's practicing physicians in America do not like the profession they are in and would not do it over again if given the chance. You do not want your child to join that group. You want success, happiness and prosperity for your child – and you can help. That is what this book is about.

If your child does decide to "become a PreMed Major" (there really is no such major), try to get accepted into medical school, then get through medical school and enter (and finish) a residency program and finally become a "real doctor' – the entire process will affect your life far more than anything else your child will ever do.

You can help, but you have to be prepared. You too will be making many sacrifices – just as your child will be entering the most competitive major on campus. Many students will not make the cut and that too will affect you as much as them. Your responsibility is to do whatever you can to help your child Win in this Game of Life called Getting Accepted into Medical School.

Thus far, you have been a big part of your child's life. Off to college they went and you thought you were done. Not so, if your child wants to become a doctor. At least it shouldn't be. Some parents slam the door shut and wish them well. So Long, Farewell, Adios, Aufweidersehen and away they go.

Unfortunately, that's probably not helping your child very much in this, the most competitive and grueling of dreams. The "premedical major" {PreMed} is filled with potholes, hurdles and an unknown host of nefarious tricksters lurking and hoping to trip up your child.

These tricksters do their job well because we simply have too many students who want to become doctors – and we will not allow that to happen! I say "we" but in fact there is no identifiable and specific person or group doing this dirty deed, it is the system which we have built and into which your child dreams of entering that does the trick.

This book is about that dream, that system, those tricks and your child.

There is much you can do. But unless you know what that "much" entails, you cannot help. Many parents do know what it takes to become a doctor. Some are doctors themselves, some were PreMed many years ago, and some just intuitively know how to succeed and have maybe already taught their child the lessons of winning, competing and getting accepted into medical school. But even then, nothing is guaranteed in the premedical world of the 21st Century.

Medical schools are drastically changing their curriculums, the students' skills and talents that formerly "got you accepted" are being modified, and the practice of medicine is far different today than it was just twenty, or even ten, years ago. This book addresses those issues as it relates to you as a parent of a PreMed Hopeful.

If you want to someday say the words, "Hello, here's my daughter the neurosurgeon," then I recommend you learn a bit about this strange and new world of PreMed. You can make a difference. You can support your child in his or her dream of becoming a doctor.

You can help your child in the courageous desire to begin an exciting journey that leads to a successful, happy and rewarding life as a practicing physician.

The best time to plant a tree is twenty years ago.

The second best time is today.

Chinese Proverb

SECTION I
SIMPLY GETTING STARTED

Who is Dr. Kapp

I'm not a college campus premedical advisor. I'm not trained in counseling psychology and I do not tell you how to raise your children. I cannot guarantee your child admission into any medical school. And lastly, I am not affiliated with any medical school. In fact, I'm not even a university professor or teacher (although I have been in the past at several prestigious universities). If that's not a confidence booster in trusting your sibling's entire career on, then I don't know what is! Why then should you consider following my advice?

Think about this for a moment. I'm someone with thousands and thousands of hours studying and researching how doctors became doctors. I've studied what makes some doctors happy and successful, while others are miserable failures – but doctors nonetheless. I've studied what it means to be competitive. I've talked with hundreds, no thousands, of doctors about what made them successful or not. I've thought about what it means to find your destiny and serve humanity through medicine. I've spent years listening to students tell me about their trials and tribulations in the PreMed World.

It turns out that my mission in life, my calling so to speak, is about helping make sure that the next generation of doctors find their mission and calling in life. Medicine is a fantastic career, but only for the right student and for the right reasons. It's not for everyone. But for the right student, and for the right reasons, it is a fantastic future awaiting their arrival.

My mission is making sure that happens. It all starts with admission to medical school. But the manner in which that occurs is not what is happening on today's college campus. Our national applicant selection process is flawed, outdated and jammed-packed with students who should have never considered medicine as a career choice in the first place.

And GUESS WHAT – That last sentence is exactly what is wrong with today's practice of medicine! It doesn't start with acceptance into medical school, it starts years earlier. Long before a student, your child, ever declares being a PreMed Major.

Over 50% of practicing physicians in America would not go into medicine again, given the choice. That sad fact reflects what is wrong with our applicant selection process. However, medicine is a fantastic profession for the right student. It is a personally and financially rewarding career available to anyone.

That was my starting point several decades ago. I repeat: It is a personally and financially rewarding career available to anyone.

I know, beyond all doubt, what works and what doesn't work. As a practicing emergency room physician for the past 30 years, I have watched doctors come and go. I went through the process; they went through the process – that being undergraduate premedical courses, medical school, post-graduate training (where you really learn what medicine is all about) and then the practice of medicine itself. Some doctors love what they do; some hate it.

I have come to the conclusion that the difference between love versus hate for our selected profession all starts long before anyone ever applies to medical school. In fact, many years before. I would argue that there is no one else on any college campus advising or coaching PreMed students who has as much worldly experience about the medical profession as me. I live and breathe medicine on a daily basis, and have been doing so for the past 30 some years.

I am not your typical campus premedical advisor. I leave the day-to-day operations to them. I am a specialist, and I specialize on not just getting your child accepted into medical school (although that too is a most important and necessary step), but also on what it really means to be a doctor and how to start thinking and acting like one now. NOW, long before applying to medical school. These two facets (acting/thinking like a doctor and acceptance) complement each other very well and the med school admissions committees take notice.

This is a paradigm shift long overdue. I believe that our crisis in medicine is largely a consequence of our doctors not understanding what they are getting into. Students are swayed by the glamour and glitz seen on TV.

Our many campus premedical advisors, as good as they are at what they do, simply do not have the background and foundation of what it really means to be a doctor. It is my belief that every parent with a child who dreams of being a doctor should read this book. Your beliefs and intentions are one thing, but the actions you and your child

11

take are another. If you have high hopes for your child, and want your actions to match those hopes, I suggest that you start by reading this book and then talk to your child about his or her exciting future.

This book was written for parents, specifically for those parents of the students I personally coach. My students are enrolled in my course, Advanced PreMed Life Support, and also spend a considerable time reading and thinking about another publication I have written, called *PreMed Pearls*.

While these stand-alone books could be studied independently, they function best when presented in a personal one-on-one coaching relationship between student and instructor. Your son or daughter as student, and myself as the instructor coach, make a powerful combination that few others can match. Working together, we develop a strategic plan directed to getting your child admitted into medical school and prepared for a happy and successful career in medicine.

While I cannot guarantee acceptance into medical school, admissions committees being unpredictable independent entities, I do provide my financial guarantee because I am so profoundly confident that my program does what I say it will do. I prepare your son or daughter to the highest standards that make admissions officers drool-with-envy when they see what they are potentially accepting.

Historically, it has been the medical school in the driver's seat of making the acceptance offer; my goal is to put your child in the driver's seat on deciding which medical school he or she decides to attend. That is an educational shift long overdue!

So let's get started and think a little about motivation. Motivation is the foundation of all success. Motivation is what will get your child that med school acceptance letter. Motivation is fuel and once you have it, it lasts a lifetime!

Does Your Child Have Internal Motivation

There is no other career that requires as many years of training as medicine before you get to start your real job. From a minimum of 11 years, and often upwards of 15 to 16 years of study and training, after high school, before you get to "know what you are doing in this business." That's a long time, a lot of tuition bills to be paid, and a thousand chances where something just might go wrong and derail the entire process.

As a parent, this is what you need to understand:

If your child isn't motivated to dedicate the effort and years required to become a doctor, then there is nothing you, I or anyone else can do that will make a difference. Success in this business comes only through effort, work and total dedication.

Did you notice what is missing in that last sentence? I didn't say that your child has to be an intellectual genius. The myth that all doctors are super-smart is just that, a myth. Of course, your child must still have the intellectual ability to memorize facts and figures, get through college courses with good grades, and take tests without freaking out, but the common societal belief that doctors have to have an IQ that borders on the genius is simply and blatantly false (more about this later).

What your child needs more than anything else in order to succeed in medicine (and this is also true in pretty much every other career choice) is a "tremendous amount of motivation" for medicine. If you know anything about college and the premedical process on campus, you know that this is exactly what is not being provided to anyone. What I do for my one-on-one coaching students is motivate them by creating a program around them that allows each student to "see the light at the end of the tunnel." They start thinking and acting like doctors now and that allows them to not just retain, but also increase their motivation for this exciting career choice.

The first step in this coaching process is based on interest. Your child must be interested in science and medicine. Do you remember your high school days? Do you remember anything from the classes that you were not interested in? The answer: Nope! Schools still teach those boring, of-no-interest classes and students the world-over still "could care less." And they learn nothing from those teachers!

On the other hand, we all took interesting classes that were so much fun that they were easy, a joy to learn about, and time just flew by. That all happened because those interesting classes generated Internal Motivation. They were interesting, you had passion for the material and everything flowed. You have undoubtedly heard the expression, "being in the flow." This mental state is what every elite performer strives for – and it all starts with Internal Motivation. Studying all those years to become a doctor is no different.

Your job as a parent is to also become a source for your child's internal motivation and fuel that fire to learn year after year after year. You don't have to be a doctor, scientist or know anything about medicine at all to be motivational fuel. But you do have to be there for emotional support, encouragement and love.

Oftentimes, many parents mistake external motivating factors for what is really needed. Examples of using errant external motivators are such things as: We'll pay you one hundred dollars to get an 'A' in that class; If you don't become a doctor, our lives are ruined; If you don't study all week, you cannot go to the party; and a thousand other ways to de-motivate anyone who ever thought about going to medical school.

External motivating factors work only in the short-term, but never in the long-term. Medicine is a marathon that takes years to complete. Your child must really, really WANT to become a doctor because he, or she, internally wants it. If your child is doing it for you, or any other outside external factor, then you have a problem.

Guess what – the money and prestige that goes with being a doctor are only external motivating factors. And now you see why over 50% of practicing physicians would not choose medicine as a career a second time. They originally made the mistake of relying on money and prestige as their motivating sources to get them through the process and now "the rooster has come home to roost" and they hate medicine – their freely chosen career.

Therefore, your goal as a supportive parent is to stoke the internal fuels of desire. My training program is also completely focused in this direction. My Advanced PreMed Life Support Course drives home those internal motivating factors so your child is coached into wanting this for himself. He unravels his (or her) own beliefs.

Together, we develop processes and tools that support the internal passion that is critical to success as a physician. Doing this now, rather than later when it is too late, makes your child stand-out in the PreMed Applicant Pool and beyond. Once we harness your child's internal engine for motivation – the rest is history, so to speak.

If you want to read more about how you can help, then continue on to the next chapter.

Ronald Kapp, MD, PhD

What's a Parent to Do

———————————~————————————

The Profession of Medicine is a team sport – doctor, nurse, tech, scribe, auditor, biller, administrator, etc. The PreMed World that your child is entering is a solo effort! At least that is how most people see it. Can you clearly see the dis-connect? The paradox of it all? And the need to radically change?

I hope so, because that is exactly my point. The profession of medicine has become a team sport for a reason. That is how we efficiently get things done. That is how we do good work. That is how we save lives.

The solo doctor is a rare zebra today. In fact, there really aren't any. A doctor may think he is in a solo-practice, but in reality he still has a receptionist, a nurse, a billing person or two, an auditor, and on-and-on. One person cannot do it all.

Why should PreMed be any different? It shouldn't be. It must not be. Many might say – but it's not, my college has a PreMed Advisor and some even have PreMed Committees. And if you think that is enough, that the advisor and committee are there specifically for your child and your child alone – well, good luck on that one! Whether it's ten, fifty, or even one hundred and fifty Premed hopefuls on campus, your school advisor or committee has a legal responsibility to treat each student equally, fairly and non-discriminatorily. And that's how it should be because that is their job.

I'm sorry, but sometimes the world's not fair. If you think that it's fair when over 300,000 freshmen students (nobody knows the exact

17

number) enter college each year thinking and maybe wanting to go to medical school and become doctors, but less than 20,000 eventually get accepted into medical school 4 years later – well, to me that is just not fair.

With all due respect to the system, perhaps many of those original students either changed their minds and found something better, didn't score high enough in their classes or on their MCAT testing session, or simply decided that a career in medicine was not for them, I am still of the opinion that the PreMed World is a Tournament. Some win, some lose. Some move on, some fall back.

Even a balanced look at the final annual PreMed applicant pool – those with 3.6 GPAs, stratospheric MCAT scores, Nobel-Peace-Prize-winning letters of evaluation, or even published research papers often do not win in the PreMed Tournament and cannot get accepted into medical school. No one says they would not make great doctors. No one says they are not qualified. What they say instead is, *"Well, sorry about that, try again next year."*

Not a very comforting thought after all that work. Pick up any medical school catalog and you will see the reality of this competitive world.

What's a Parent to Do? We all want what is best for our children, but few know what to do. Few parents keep up with this changing PreMed World. We leave it up to our one lone child who goes off to college, eager, hopeful and wanting to become a doctor and hope for the best.

As we all know, hope is not a good strategy for success (outside the lottery system that is).

For students to make progress in this competitive PreMed World, they must want to study and do well, have a high level of Internal Motivation, and be receptive to developing a Comprehensive PreMed Team (more about this later).

In reality, there are really only two types of students on any college campus:

(1) The Internally Motivated who get their work done by being interested, attentive, caring and dedicated.

(2) The Externally Motivated who study and work only when something drives them in the short-term.

The Internally Motivated students are easy to work with and they seem to always make fantastic progress. They set the bar for others to follow.

The Externally Motivated, on the other hand, are always a struggle from day one. After more than 20 years of studying what's makes a good doctor good, I have come to the conclusion that nearly every Externally Motivated person has the same root cause. In medicine we name it the etiologic factor that drives behavior.

I have found that the Externally Motivated are a product of their parents' attempts at discipline and motivation at a very early age. (In fact, this is standard psychological theory regarding behavior.) Parents often push their children out of love and a caring desire for wanting them to excel – which carries over into adulthood as an Externally Motivated behavior pattern. Obviously this does not work well in the competitive, long and grueling PreMed Tournament.

The self-motivated win in the PreMed Tournament; the externally-motivated lose. A rather simple dichotomy. In reality it takes much more than simply being self-motivated to get accepted into medical school, but these students are much easier to work with, have a higher acceptance rate and eventually make far better and more successful doctors.

Here's the tough part: Externally Motivated students frequently do not know they are that way. Their beliefs are hidden. Often times they do not even know that they are working to serve someone else's interests.

Many do not realize that they are going to college to please someone else. They cannot see that their choice of a "doctor career" is more important to someone else, rather than themselves.

Many of the Externally Motivated students have never examined why they do what they do, why they want what they want, or who wants what for anything in life.

Many of these students still get accepted into medical school, graduate and become doctors, and later – often many years later – find that medicine is not what they should have chosen as a career. This may be one of life's greatest preventable tragedies.

The key to unraveling this mystery of choice is understanding. Every student must come to grips with why he, or she, wants to go to college, study for years and become a doctor. Each student is a unique individual who must deeply examine their personal beliefs of why certain behaviors exist or do not exist. Believe me, colleges don't do this for you. Professors don't have the time.

There is no one on campus who even wants to begin this unraveling-of-beliefs to examine why your son or daughter thinks medicine is a good career choice.

As a parent, you can begin the process at home. Long before your offspring ever enters college. You can, and should, be the first member of your child's PreMed Team. Communication is key. (Yes, I know, who communicates these days?) You must sit down with your child and start asking questions.

Find out what he or she wants out of life. Don't worry, it will change. Often too. Your goal is to listen, not lecture. Your goal is to guide, not direct. What you offer is loving support for what your child wants, not for what you want. Easier said than done, but it has to start today. The sooner the better and the more the better.

Another way of looking at this process is as if you are starting to build your Personal PreMed Team. Remember, medicine is a team sport. You and your child are the beginning of a team. Together you can begin the process of trying to figure out life.

But always remember – you are not a dictator, you are not an oppressor, you are there as a parental guide and source of loving support.

Think about this for a moment.

Which will Internally Motivate your child more – *"I've decided you should go to medical school and become a doctor!"* OR ... *"Tell me what excites and drives you and what might you want to do with your life?"* Pretty obvious when you look at life this way.

The key to success is to focus on what your child wants, not what you want. Let your child know that you are there for support when needed. Let them know that your years of experience and wisdom mean something, but not everything.

There's an old joke that goes something like this: The student says, *"Boy, when I was 16 it was amazing how stupid my parents were. But now, only 5 years later, it's even more amazing how much they learned in the last 5 years."*

PreMed is a world unto itself. The most competitive major on campus. The hardest classes of any. The lowest probability of success of any. And your child enters this world alone and hoping for the best. It's up to you to give them every chance to succeed and become what he or she wants to become. The choice is yours. The choice is theirs.

21

Together, as a team, you can enter the PreMed Tournament seeded higher than your neighbor and with a far better chance of success.

Clarity is power and the best way to make your child want to study and learn anything is to open a clear path in his head that effort today leads to the ultimate goals that he, and only he, wants (unless of course, he is a she).

Your job as a parental team-mate is to assist in this goal of developing clarity for your child. There are many others who will help along the way, but you will always remain primary. It is a heavy responsibility, but medicine is a rewarding 40 year career for those who undertake the journey.

What you, as a parent, can do now:

- Come to grips with the fact that this is your child's career. Until you realize this truth, no real progress will ever be made.

- Your goal is to guide your child, but not lead. Pushing, telling, demanding will never help. Your child has to really, really want to be a doctor.

- Schedule a time now to sit down with your child and ask what he or she wants out of life. Your goal is to primarily listen. Let your child begin the process of discovery. Let him (or her) know that you are there whenever needed to simply listen and act as a sounding-board.

- Ask what specific "tangible things" he might want in life. Tangibles such as money, cars, house, boat, family, etc.

- Then ask what specific "intangible things" he might want in life. Intangibles such as respect, satisfaction, love, feeling of accomplishment, etc.

- Make a written list of the "tangible" and the "intangible" desires of your child from the above two questions. This will really focus your child and also show that you are listening and care.

- Repeat this entire process on a regular schedule (maybe every other month or so) to see how your child's thoughts and desires might change (or not).

Ronald Kapp, MD, PhD

Know Thy Child, Know Thy Schools

When we are first born, we all have essentially the same potential. At that point we don't know who is intelligent, who might be athletic, or who might be talented in art, music or even history. We definitely do not know who will or will not make a good doctor! A question I have been addressing for many years is "when do we know when someone will make a good doctor?"

It turns out that we really don't know the answer to that question until many years later, typically after they become a doctor. Whoa, do you see the problem now?

Here is how our current "PreMed Selection Process" works: We are asking your 18 year old child when he enters college – do you want to be a doctor? Then, 4 years later we "choose" those students with the highest GPA and MCAT scores to attend our medical schools. That's the entire process.

Now there may be a few variations from campus to campus, but basically this is a "get on the train now" sort of system. While we may debate the fine points of my opinion – the underlying truth is that certain courses must be taken (the typical campus premedical course requirements) and you better get an 'A' and while you're at it you should add in a few letters of recommendation too, and maybe a project or two also, and maybe a sport or something political or perhaps something humanitarian or maybe you should just publish a book or two to stand out a little more.

You get the point I hope. It's competitive.

I am a firm believer in competition and the American way of fighting your way to the top. Winner-take-all is my motto. If you can't make it, too bad – so sad. In fact, that's a pretty good belief system in our current PreMed World of "get your GPA and MCAT scores as high as you can." Unfortunately, that also leads to a lot of unhappy future doctors.

However, there is a solution – "Know Thy Child, Know Thy Schools."

Your child probably doesn't know what college is like – how could he since he hasn't been there yet. Unless you have been to medical school yourself, neither of you know much or anything about that either. Residency presents the same conundrum. And practicing as a doctor is a totally unknown territory for even many of us still working in the profession!

And yet there is a solution – Know Thy Child, Know Thy Schools.

I choose Ohio State University. A large school with a lot of opportunity. I went to graduate school at UT-Austin, another large behemoth of an institution. I then attended UT- Houston Medical School (not a small place by any means). At the time, these seemed to fit my personality. I was offered opportunity and programs unimaginable on smaller campuses. I could study and also remain anonymous. It worked for me, at the time.

Many of my friends choose smaller schools. Much smaller. I'm quite certain they too were pleased with their selections, at the time. Hopefully it worked out well for them also. My high school graduating class of about 300 students probably went to 100 different campuses.

From that small suburb in Cleveland, we populated campuses of all types across the country. The question I have asked myself over and over is: "How did we know?" The answer to this philosophical question is: "We didn't, we took a flying leap."

Now, many years later, I realize that taking a flying leap is not a very good strategy. A far better strategy would have been to try much harder to understand myself, try to understand who I am as a person and what and why I believe as I do, and then address what I want out of life and what legacy might I want to leave behind. Heavy questions for anyone; and especially heavy for a 16 or 18 or 20 or even 22 year old child.

So it boils down to either (1) taking a flying leap or (2) trying to understand yourself. Medicine is a full-time profession, typically allowing 40 years or more for practicing that profession, and maybe generating hundreds of thousands of dollars income every year.

It also takes a lot of work and a lot of years before that income ever starts returning to your bank account. Not to mention the simple truth that only a handful of hopefuls even get accepted after their 4 years of undergraduate premedical preparation.

This all leads to the second part of my quote above – Know Thy Schools. It is critical to match your school choice with what you want and who you are as a person. Small fish, big pond; big fish, small pond. Each offers benefits. Each has disadvantages. Individual instruction and small classes might be nice. The personal touch of a small, private institution is often welcomed. On the other hand, divergent opportunities on the behemoth campus can also be rewarding.

Unless you know yourself and understand your beliefs, you cannot make an informed decision. And it is only through informed decisions and choices that anyone can make the best of their God-given potential.

The point is that you have to know a little about yourself and a little about the schools you hope to attend. This is where parents often play a pivotal role in helping get their child on the train to success. Parental feedback is critical. Parents know their children better than anyone. In fact, this is such an important factor that I have even developed a feedback section in my Advanced PreMed Life Support Course for this very purpose.

Over the years, I have found that knowing how to give and receive feedback, while not well known to most, is critically important in modeling behavior, in climbing the ladder of success, and even in getting accepted into medical school.

We are often instructed on how to give feedback, but it turns out that knowing how to receive feedback is even more important. I have learned that it is often these simple things that make a profound difference in how we turn out and what we make of our lives.

The matching of child personality to type of institution is an often neglected component in our decisions of what to do and when to do it. Being a PreMed Major does not afford such neglect. That PreMed Train runs fast and furious, and you definitely want the right seat if possible.

How I Work

If you have read my book this far it is obvious that you are serious about turning your child into a doctor. Many might offer the opinion that this should best be left up to our universities and medical schools. I whole-heartedly disagree with that advice on a number of accounts:

The typical undergraduate university faculties are trained as Ph.D.'s and not Medical Doctors. They have neither the fundamental understanding, nor the proper clinical training to properly prepare future doctors. Nor do they have the time and rarely the interest.

College is a time of competition and weeding out of the not-qualified-as-doctor material via the PreMed Tournament format.

There are many, many PreMed hopefuls on every college campus who receive rejection letter after rejection letter, but would make fantastic physicians if given the chance.

Medical schools themselves are far too busy teaching the technical knowledge base of medicine at the obvious detriment of leaving out the personal touches of what makes for a great physician. They all hope this happens by simple osmosis – a fact that over 50% of practicing physicians today most likely missed out on.

Medical schools are homogenous pots of high scoring GPA-MCAT students, still focused on individual effort and gain. There is little room for learning how to be a doctor and how to be part of a team.

Ronald Kapp, MD, PhD

Residency programs, notwithstanding the fact that slave-labor still exists, are primarily a "model me behavior" system that perpetuates the status quo.

I suppose that every point above could be debated ad-nauseum, but the fact remains that the best time to begin the process of trying to understand who we are as individuals and what we want out of life should be as early and as soon as possible. That PreMed Train that your child is hoping to board is a fast-running machine that is both hard-to-get-on and also hard-to-get-off.

Therefore, what I have developed is an online course (*Advanced PreMed Life Support*) that addresses the main issues of (1) why, how, when, where and what should a PreMed student do and think about in order to make that informed decision – should I become a doctor or not and if I do decide to do it – (2) what should I be doing to maximize my opportunity for success.

My goal is to get students to see the light at the end of the tunnel. This definitely enhances their internal motivation and adds fuel to their drive to succeed.

My analogy is this: Every elite athlete and sporting team (on campus and off) utilize coaches to maximize their effort. Most even use a team of coaches and assistant coaches in order to win. Why is PreMed treated so differently?

Furthermore: If you wanted to learn how to fly an airplane, would you not seek out a pilot? Or if you wanted to learn how to play professional tennis, would not a tennis pro be best?

Why is PreMed treated so differently? And who best to select?

Advanced PreMed Life Support is a specialized program for elite students. You do not need to be a genius to be a good doctor, but you do need access to and training by someone who knows what the

30

profession of medicine is all about. Campus advisors are generalists who treat all students equally. To excel in anything, you need a specialist.

Therefore, I created a unique, proprietary program with the following goals in mind:

- Unravel the underlying belief system of each individual student regarding his or her wants and desires of why medicine is my destiny.

- Develop a unique personal profile, a blueprint for success, which maximizes the chances of winning in the PreMed Tournament.

- Begin the process of thinking and acting like the future physician you want to be.

- Development of a fund of knowledge that is medicine-based and useful in the PreMed process.

- Introduction to the reality of medicine on what your future is going to be like.

The **APLS** Course is delivered online in an inter-active fashion. Students have direct access to me via SKYPE and email. This course is not difficult, but it can be intense. Together, your child and I begin the unraveling process of why beliefs are as they are and what we can do about it.

This can unearth some heavy baggage for some students. However, I believe it is better to figure this out now, long before years and years of effort and thousands of dollars have been invested in the PreMed Hope of winning in the tournament, but losing because some little artifact of hindrance was left unsaid, uncovered and undiscovered.

31

However, I am neither psychologist nor psychiatrist and leave that domain to those professionals. I simple put forth the questions and query what every student should want to know about themselves and the profession and how to go about winning the tournament and getting an acceptance letter into medical school.

The online **APLS** format is non-threatening and allows any student to decline responses whenever so desired. There is no grade and there is no pressure for a correct answer. All answers are correct, some are just better than others. My goal is to assist each student in finding his or her best answer.

No college credit is given for taking this course, but the end-result may turn out to be the best college course your child has ever taken.

Due to the interactive nature of this course and how much time I must personally devote to each student, I can only accept a limited number of students each year. A student may devote as much or as little time and effort, but understand that you only get out as much as you put in.

There is no magic in gaining acceptance into medical school. It takes work, effort and a full-time dedication that no other major on campus requires.

However, it remains my fervent belief that almost anyone has the intellectual capability to master the profession of medicine and become a successful, happy and great doctor. It just takes a little coaching by the right person at the right time under the right circumstances to Win The PreMed Tournament.

When you sign up for the **APLS** course, your child will work directly with me. It is a course I have been perfecting for over 20 years. If you decide to enroll your child in this course, know in advance that this will be an intense process. It is only offered to students who want to understand themselves and who are willing to dedicate the effort to seriously think about the questions before they answer.

My response at times, like those of any good coach, may not be to you or to your child's liking. I believe that is how it should be. I am coaching for winning results, not to win a popularity contest.

I'm easy to get along with and pleasant to work with, and I always keep an upbeat, positive mood – but I also know that someone (probably you) paid me a lot of money for this course so I do not spoon-feed anyone. Your child has to want this. They have to work. They must put in the effort. If I detect a lack-of-effort or that it's just-not-working for them or me, I pro-rate all fees and refund un-used portions as I send your child back to their campus premedical advisor(s) and wish both the best of luck.

My mission is coaching the future doctors of America who want and believe in medicine as a calling and destiny. Together we are bound to **Solve Our Health Care Crisis, One Doctor at a Time**. With your help, with your child, I know we can do it.

Ronald Kapp, MD, PhD

SECTION II
THE FOUNDATIONS OF BEING
A PREMED PARENT

How Important are the Undergraduate PreMed Years?

That question is a little like asking, "How important is air?" I approach everything done before medical school acceptance (BMSA) as critically important to becoming a doctor. That even includes effort during high school years – although no one will ever look at what happened then, unless it was really bad like getting arrested or being a terrorist. No one cares about your high school grades or your SAT score – those are just the things that got you into college.

It's the college years that count. Unfortunately, it was all the effort and work you did in high school that prepares you for college and if you enter college unprepared then you are already at the end of the PreMed line waiting to board that fast-moving train. In other words, you cannot afford to be unprepared for college.

PreMed starts on Day One.

Nobody in college will tell you this, and many advisors might not even agree with this, but it is the reality of choosing the toughest major on campus. Some might tell you, *"Don't worry about that low grade in Freshman English. They only look at your science grades."* While that may be technically somewhat correct (to a point), the medical school admissions committees are still made up of real people making real decisions, and if you think they are going to ignore that low grade because you were *"just getting warmed up"* then you do not understand the competitive world your child has just entered.

Here's my analogy: Imagine you just got a new job. You show up for work on the very first day, but you were late and didn't take the time to put on some nice clothes. When your boss looks at you like you just got off a boat from China, you respond with, *"Gee, it's only the first day."* How do you think you now compare to all the other first day hires and how long do you think you'll last in that job?

Being PreMed is even more extreme than that. The impression you make and the grades you get from Day One follow you like a shadow.

I look at PreMed as "climbing the ladder of success." That is what it really is! It's no different than being hired at a large corporation as an intern in the mail room and eventually working your way up to being the VP of Finance. Only in this case, your child is judged by a very specific set of premedical criteria that have little or nothing to do with being a doctor, but all of which must be done to get you there.

Sure, mistakes along the way (like low grades) can be overcome, or really bad days (like bombing the MCAT) can be forgotten, but the effort to overcome these basic types of mistakes takes a herculean

36

effort and sometimes extra years of work. There are a lot of mail room interns wanting to become a VP, and there are even more undergraduate students wanting to become a doctor. Many of those competitors began their climb during their early years of high school and arrive into college prepped and ready to go!

If all this sounds a bit stressful and over-the-top as you think about the potential competition, you should realize that it is. It doesn't have to be that way. It does not have to be stressful and approached in a do-or-die fashion.

I wanted to make that point because that is how many do approach their PreMed career. They look at PreMed as a "one-shot chance" to get accepted. But that's not the case. That's how the schools might want your child to play it, but it doesn't have to be that way. In fact, it shouldn't be played that way.

Your child may change his or her mind about even wanting to become a doctor. He might be better suited for something else. She might be happier in a different career. Both might find the Game of PreMed just a bit ridiculous.

Many students quit the PreMed race as soon as they see the requirements and hurdles before them. It's sort of like looking up at Mt. Everest from base camp and thinking, *"I have to climb that sucker!"*

Fortunately, there are alternative approaches to successfully getting through the PreMed process and that is what the **APLS** Course is all about. I still maintain that this is a most serious endeavor and must be approached that way, but it need not be stressful and a win-at-all-cost battle.

Students just need to be coached and guided in the right way so that they understand why they are doing certain things, what activities they should be doing or not doing, and when they should "charge up that hill" or "retreat." If the coach wants your team to win the National Championship or the Super Bowl, the players had better understand why certain things are done or not done. It's that simple.

Simple that is if you already know all about medicine and how to navigate the process. Complicated if you don't. Therein lies the rub – how can you expect your son or daughter to know these things as they leave home, some for the first time in their life, and enter that PreMed pool. It's a deep pool with no bottom for many. Sink or swim is not a good strategy for success.

But that's where you come in. Even though you may not be in college and may be hundreds or thousands of miles away, you can still be there in heart and spirit – and that means a lot to someone trying to solve this riddle of acceptance.

It is an obvious fact that all undergraduate grades are important. It is also a fact that science grades in upper division classes are even more important. Your child will arrive on campus and one of the first things he will hear is how important the GPA (grade point average) and the MCAT (medical college admissions test) scores are to getting accepted into medical school.

It seems like almost everyone boasts how great their students are, either as undergraduates or as entering medical school classes, by pointing to that coveted GPA and MCAT. Yes, there is reality to that boast – although a sad reality it is. There is little to no correlation between GPA/MCAT scores and future physician quality. That's right – the GPA means nothing. No patient, hospital or clinic has ever asked me what my GPA was. Most don't even know what MCAT stands for.

However, that is the focus of campus premedical advisors and even most medical school admissions committees. These scores open the door to success. But these alone are not enough. There are thousands upon thousands upon thousands of PreMed applicants with cosmic grades and MCATs. In fact, with a little planning, taking the right courses at the right time, a little coaching and some serious study, I believe your son and daughter, even those of average intelligence, can most likely join that high GPA club.

A lot of people don't like it when I say what I just said, even those of average intelligence. But it's true. Getting high PreMed grades is more of a game than anything. I guarantee that your campus premedical advisor is not going to be showing your son or daughter the ropes on how it's done. That person (or committee) needs to treat everyone as an equal.

However, we are not equal – your goal is to get an acceptance letter and not a rejection letter. You can best do that by outscoring your fellow students. And doing a few other things. That alone makes this an unequal playing field – sort of like life itself.

It's those few other things that often make the difference. You cannot just study, study, study and get those grades and hope to get accepted. And you would not want to. Although many do, those students later find out that medicine is far different that what they thought it would be. Their tunnel vision may have led to short-term success, but guaranteed long-term failure.

Their college years were not put to good use. Those 3 or 4 years are critically important. Not simply for grades and MCAT scores that get your child accepted, but for a whole host of other reasons, such as:

- Developing Good Study Habits

- Learning Time Management Skills

- Dealing with Daily Stress

- Overcoming Exam Anxiety

- Learning How to Take Tests

- Discovering How to Handle Uncertainty

- Mastering Fear of Success, & Sometimes Failure

- Learning How to Prioritize the Important from the Mundane

- Understanding Personal Emotions

- Discovering a Personal Identity

- Controlling the Party Animal Within

- Being a Leader & a Team Player

- Realizing that Persistence Wins the Tournament

- Having the Courage to Change Direction if Necessary

- Practicing Humility

- Realizing that Listening is More Important than Talking

- Developing Empathy

- Learning How to Think & Act Like a Doctor

- Discovering Inner Passion

- Growing Up and Learning What Life is About

All those and even a few more go into what the college years are all about. And those things are not learned if all your child ever does is study, study, study.

Don't get me wrong here; studying is critically important and your child will become a studying-monster and a test-taking-machine, but even more is needed to win in this competitive PreMed World. No team wins a National Championship without a lot of hard work and some luck along the way, becoming a doctor is lot like that too. But the satisfaction of both lasts a long, long time.

That being said, I think most will agree that the undergraduate college years are pretty darn important. I talk with a lot of older students who often lament that they wasted their time in college, but now many years later still have that inner-pulling of desire that being a doctor is something they still want to do.

Wasted years can be overcome, but it takes some extra hard work and dedication to prove yourself worthy over those 20 year old maniacal, test-taking-machines that boarded that train right at the starting line from Day One.

Some students just seem to know right from the start on what to do and how to do it. Maybe their parents are doctors, or someone in the family told them what to do, or maybe their friends clued them in on how competitive this race really is – but somehow they just knew. That gives them a big advantage.

Some students even took the extra time to take speed-reading classes while in high school (I did). If there is one thing that gives any student a tremendous advantage in winning this tournament – that would be it.

The amount of material a PreMed student is exposed to and has to master is gargantuan and speed-reading is one essential tool for that competitive advantage.

It's my opinion that the second most important tool for any PreMed student to have is knowing how to memorize. Knowing how to memorize facts, tables, and useless formulas. This is a teachable and trainable skill.

I know of few high schools that specifically teach this skill, and yet right along with speed-reading, these two skills make up the most potent one-two punch in getting accepted into medical school (and

Ronald Kapp, MD, PhD

help even more in getting through) than anything else any student can ever do. No one teaches this, students rarely study these skills and yet those who do somehow possess these two tools – and tools they are – are always leading the pack. These are two of the intangible skills that nobody talks about, but when you have them in your armamentarium – yes, big words are the third skill that successful students possess!

An impressive vocabulary is right there at the top of my list of tools that every student must possess. Doctors use big words. In fact, what really makes doctoring seem so special is our unique and specialized vocabulary. *The underlying etiology of that patient's idiopathic thrombocytopenia purpura remains a puzzling enigma to his hematologist.*

 Hopefully your son or daughter won't take it to that extreme, but you should get the point that a prolific elocution might just help your offspring edge out another student without such a skill.

I have the unique ability of simply listening to someone speak for a few minutes and knowing their educational level. I listen to the words they use. I listen to their grammar. I evaluate their sentence construction. I instinctually unravel their thought processes. My end result: I knew their educational level and can sometimes even guess their profession. And if you think this is a unique ability to me – then you do not know medical school admissions committees and how they work!

A personal interview is still a required step in the application process into medical school. While this is usually a moot point for most good students, it does sometimes make or break the case.

Those interviewers are listening to your child speak – words, grammar, sentence construction, thought processes, etc that make up an eloquent and intelligent speaker are being evaluated – sometimes not even on a conscious level by the interviewer. My point: Basic undergraduate

SECTION II – How Important are the Undergraduate Years?

English classes are extremely important in getting your son or daughter accepted into medical school. *Who wudda thunk it!*

In summary, here's what college (or even better yet, what should have been learned-high-school-skills) should teach your child:

- Speed-Reading

- Memorization Skills

- Vocabulary

- English Grammar

I call those the Big-4 Skills that help your child get though college with good grades, get accepted into medical school and impress the day-lights out of their future patients after they become doctors. This is not rocket-science, it is simply fundamental education that is often neglected.

However, in this arena of being a PreMed major and entering the PreMed Tournament that not everyone wins, these tools (simply learned skills) often make a tremendous difference between acceptance and rejection.

Those undergraduate years are critically important in learning these skills. There will be no time later in life to go back and learn how to read, speak, and think.

I will defend our current premedical application process a little here by saying that the student with a high GPA and fantastic MCAT scores probably knows and practices these skills far better than a student who scores much lower, but that is not always the case. Courses can be gamed.

MCAT review courses can probably prep a monkey to score pretty well on the MCAT. And a half-way intelligent student can get through a personal interview by not saying much. In other words, some doctors still end up un-educated and unable to effectively communicate with their patients – so they become orthopedic surgeons – NO, just kidding!

Don't get all worried and stressed out if your child still reads, speaks and thinks like the typical California teenager – have you been out there lately – because much of this is like that old chicken-and-egg question of which came first.

Education is a holistic endeavor. In other words, it will all happen together as your child takes various courses and puts two and two together.

We have a joke in medicine – PreMed and medical students are kept in the dark for years, we feed them crap year after year, and eventually they come out as mushrooms – a fine delicacy known as a doctor. The spores of that mushroom must be planted during your child's undergraduate years and preferably before.

As a parent, you can encourage these skills. You could possibly invest in extra-curricular speed-reading classes. You can correct bad grammar when you hear it. You can bring books home for your child to read. You can play memory games. There's a lot you can do to help and encourage your child in learning these most-boring of skills.

They may be boring to the typical teenager, but they also make the difference between an elite accepted PreMed versus the also-ran.

Yes, crucify me now, but I'm promoting more education and more competition. As if we weren't competitive enough and I'm suggesting that the average PreMed study even more.

However, that's a debatable point. I'm suggesting that you encourage your son or daughter to learn skills that can be used as tools. Reading, speaking, and thinking are learned skills. These are life-long skills that will be valuable in any career and since doctoring is a 40 year long career, it seems logical to me that learning them now will pay tremendous dividends later.

These are not wasted skills like learning calculus or physics (although those too have a prominent place in training the brain). These are skills that make for success in all fields. Some even go so far as to say that a successful and rewarding life is dependent on the use of these skills.

Ronald Kapp, MD, PhD

How Important is Passion to a PreMed?

The fuel for the human cell is ATP (adenosine triphosphate). We get that from the food we eat. The fuel for a successful PreMed Career is Passion! Passion is that internal motivating force that drives everything your child does. The child who is passionate about baseball will go out and play that all day long. The true tennis aficionado will hit a thousand practice serves in the hope of one future ace in a match. The professional football player has hit a tackling dummy a million times or more. Passion for a PreMed student should be the same. Only usually it's not.

PreMed passion is intangible. It can't be measured. It's hard to practice. It's even hard to define and talk about:

"Gee, Mom, I want to be a doctor."

"Why?" you ask.

"I don't know. I guess because they make a lot of money."

"Oh, you don't really want a lot of money do you?"

"No, not really, I just want to help people."

That is pretty darn intangible to me. Making money seems to always be another elephant in the room that no one wants to acknowledge. Helping people sounds great, but it doesn't mean anything. And that's the problem with "even thinking about becoming a doctor." A pound of gold, a ton of effort and 10 years or more of your child's life for just thinking about wanting to become a doctor. That about sums it up for most.

I didn't know what I was getting into. I was living in a college dorm and a guy down the hall was PreMed. I thought to myself, *"I'm as smart as him; I'll be a doctor too."* That was totally wrong. Wrong in every sense of the word. Wrong in my thought process. Wrong in my decision. Just plain wrong. And yet that is how I did it.

I went to school. I got the grades. I applied. They accepted me because of my grades. No one, not one person ever asked me about my passion. **Passion?** What does that have to do with being a doctor?

It's a little better today, but not much. They ask about passion because everyone now knows how important that is, but the answers are as feeble as long ago. We don't study passion. We don't practice passion. We don't even think passion. Yet, passion remains the fuel to success.

A decade of studying and four more decades dedicated to something we knew little to nothing about. Stop a moment and think about what that means for your child. FIFTY years doing something that your child may or may not have any passion for! And we, meaning most parents and college advisors, allow your child to make this momentous decision alone, without much input or fore-thought.

That is a parenting gap that needs to be closed. But if you're not a successful, happy practicing doctor who wants to interact with your child and close that gap – what's a parent to do? What's anyone to do?

How Important is Passion to a PreMed is the question I ask every student I coach. It's even more important than the Big-4 skills that I just talked about. Passion drives those skills. It's passion that drives everything we do. Passion and love for doing what we are doing. Do

48

what you love, and love what you do. Unfortunately, easier said than done.

That's where you, the parent, come in. You have a critical role to play in this. Every child looks to you for advice, encouragement and acknowledgement. That's how we learned to walk and talk, play sports, exhibit good manners, etc.

Parental influence is powerful and of immeasurable importance. I got lucky because my parents excelled in this area. They brought out and encouraged my passion. They understood my passion. They were passionate about my passion. But, sadly, not all parents are like mine.

In fact, many parents discourage passion. They tell their child how much work it is to become a doctor, how long it takes, and how demanding the job is.

Here's the real point. Your beliefs, your wants and desires, are not your child's. Your child is a new, independent, separate-from-you, person who has his or her own passions, wants and desires. I hope that in today's enlightened world that most parents already know this, but the facts often speak differently.

Even parents who do know this simple truth are often blinded by their subconscious wants and desires. What parent would not want his or her child to be a successful, happy doctor?

Therefore, it is the truly conscious parent who stokes the flames of passion in his (her) child based on what the child wants out of life, not on what the parent wants for the child. Is it any wonder that more than 50% of today's practicing docs would not choose the same career a second time around?

Yes, your parental influence is super critical, but only if unbiased and unidirectional. That is often a tough nut to crack, but it has to be cracked nonetheless.

So that brings up full-circle back to "passion in your child" and whether or not he/she has that internal passion for wanting to become a doctor. My best analogy is similar to that of the difference between infatuation and love.

Being infatuated with someone is one thing, being in love with someone is quite another. Do you remember when you were in high school and sitting in the next row was that super-wonderful, good-looking, could-never-do-anything-wrong person? Until you got to know him and found out what a slob he (or she) was. That was infatuation. Wonderful and fantastic until you found out the true facts. Then it was a quick adios.

Infatuation rarely lasts and that's why so many of our doctors today would not choose their doctoring profession a second time. On the other hand, those doctors who found love in their profession really stick it out and enjoy what they do. Just like love, it's not always perfect and rosy but you still take the good with the bad.

Medicine is truly a marriage between person and profession. You work to fix problems, you accept what cannot be changed, you over-look obvious faults, but deep down you know that this love for medicine is your true destiny and calling. It is why you exist. It makes you complete. Might sound corny, but that is how it should be. Those doctors become successful, happy physicians.

You are probably just like me thinking, *"Sounds great, but how can that ever happen?"* Well it doesn't on most college campuses.

Today's PreMed application and selection process is sort of like being forced into marrying the first person you ever dated. It might work out, but more often it takes years of dating and being exposed to different people's personalities to see what you want in a mate, a partner for life, someone to spend the next 50 years with. That's how you find true love. It might be your high school sweetheart, but that's a rare and uniquely lucky way of finding your soul-mate.

Today's college PreMed applicant is more infatuated with the profession of medicine than being in love with it. They are infatuated with the image of the doctor on TV who saves the critically ill child with a stroke of genius. They are infatuated with the mansion and fancy cars that the media portray all doctors as having. They are infatuated with the idea of "they will come to me with all their problems and I will help everyone."

It's an infatuation that leads to a disenchanted future. A dark future of drudgery and discontent. A future wanting-of-divorce, but being unable to ever release yourself from the chains of a career that once infatuated you, but clings now as a burden of being-stuck-here-after-all-that-work.

I painted a pretty ugly picture there on purpose. For some doctors it might be that bad, but usually it's more like that dis-contented marriage that you hope will get better, but rarely does. You stick it out. You put up with it. BUT, it is my opinion that neither marriage, nor a career as a doctor should be that way. Both should be fantastic and fun. And they are if you are in love.

If you love who you are with, or love what you are doing – your future is fun and exciting. There will be problems in both, but problems that you will tackle head-on, with energy and passion. That is what you want for your mate, and that is what your child should want with his or her career.

Great, I bet we all agree! Even campus administrators and advisors would probably agree with that. A world of sweet-smelling roses all around. And that cheerful campus advisor who is taking all your tuition money as fast as you can dish it out would then ask, *"But how can that be done with all the courses that need to be taken?"* They will say, *"And we have a lot to teach your child, so you better get started right away, you don't want to miss out do you?"*

If you think about it, it all sounds a little like that used-car salesman you once met, *"You just gotta buy this one today, it'll be gone tomorrow. You just love it don't ya!"* Once again, a substitution of love for what is really just infatuation.

A career for any child should be based on far more than simple infatuation. Especially a career that takes 10 to 15 years of work just to get that first paycheck. A career that you cannot back out of demands passion, a keen sense of what you are getting into, and perhaps even love for the profession.

I am sure that it is now quite obvious to most readers that the only way to accomplish this searching for a career-I-love is through practical experience. You will not find that on many college campuses.

Practical experience only comes through being exposed to the reality of what doctors do day-after-day.

Exposure in a real clinical setting. Exposure to patients and a little of what it's like being a doctor. Practical experience of showing up at a clinic or hospital and seeing medicine being practiced by real people on real people. That will develop more passion than watching TV or reading a magazine article on doctoring. Real passion from the heart. Passion that drives behavior. Passion that lasts.

The good news is that many college campuses now have clinical shadowing experiences for their PreMed students. They send their students out into the community.

Not only do the students discover their true passion (although many don't), but the medical school admissions committees understand the long-lasting personal benefits that each student then brings with him or her into their future. It becomes a win-win for everyone.

Opportunities such as weekend or evening shadowing, week-long vacation programs, or even semester-long medical missions to foreign countries all provide a wealth of data that help your child discover an inner passion for medicine. Time spend and invested in such endeavors will pay dividends far more than you ever imagined.

That discovered inner passion will act as a fuel for continuing on, studying late at night, or overcoming any hurdle that at first seems insurmountable. Being PreMed is a career of delayed gratification.

While all your child's friends are out working and making money, your child will be hitting-the-books, studying for another test, prepping for some presentation – all of which become so much easier when your child knows and understands that his or her inner passion is the fuel for it all.

Passion makes for success. Clarity of passion creates an unstoppable force. Living your passion makes life fun, even when bad things are happening all around you.

If our practicing physicians of tomorrow discover their passion today, our health care crisis today will become the practice of medicine tomorrow that everyone wants and dreams about.

The passion of your child can make that dream a reality, rather than the nightmare it is today for so many of our country's doctors. Your child's dream of the future rests on a foundation of passion.

You can help your child uncover that passion. You may or may not know much about medicine, but you know your child and you have worldly experiences that can be put to good use.

You can, should and must be a supporting member of your child's team. There are right and wrong ways to go about doing that, and that is what Section III is about.

Ronald Kapp, MD, PhD

Your Child's Greatest Asset

Her brains? His looks? Obviously the future doctor has to look and act the part, but your child's greatest asset is YOU! You, far more than you know, play a crucial role is the entire process of getting your child accepted into medical school. Parental influence and approval are powerful forces that affect your child.

No matter your current relationship with your child, there is either one of two reasons you matter – (1) your child wants to succeed in order to prove you right, or (2) to prove you wrong.

Most parents want their children to be successful and have a great career, but interestingly some don't. Some parents believe, for a variety of reasons, that their child should not succeed, should not go to medical school and should not become a doctor. The underlying reasons for either belief are unique and varied for each family unit.

However, in order to help your child, these reasons need to be uncovered and openly discussed. Again, this discussion can go either way – sometimes it becomes a loving and wonderful experience, whereas sometimes it is rather painful and upsetting. Nonetheless, it needs to be done.

Your child is contemplating a tremendous personal journey into the unknown (doctoring) and knowledge about your family's beliefs is crucial. Do you recall the concept of "internal motivation" that I discussed earlier and how important it is to have a strong internal motivating force? The dynamics of your family unit play into this concept.

If your child (boy or girl) knows in his heart that you truly believe in his ability, intelligence and drive to succeed, he will do everything in his power to make that happen. He is doing it for a variety of subconsciously-driven psychological beliefs, all of which attempt to please you, the parent. Although this may sound a bit like external motivation (and sometimes it is), the force still arises within your child.

On the other hand, some children have a drive to succeed in order to prove their parents wrong. These children have been told, sometimes over and over for years, that they will never amount to anything and are destined for failure. These kids want to just prove you oh so wrong! Another seemingly external motivator that is internally-driven.

Of course the best of all worlds is when your child has your love and support, has been told over and over that he (and she) can become anything he sets his mind on and works to accomplish. This internal drive has been nurtured over many years of familial support. Each accomplishment in life has been a milestone and also a stepping stone to the next.

Failures, when they occur, and they must, are not discouraging events, but are used as times-for-learning. Surprisingly, this romantic notion of life-as-it-should-be is more common then you know.

There are many families out there that function this way. If yours is one of them, great. But if not, then you have a slight handicap in overcoming your past. It's not a fatal short-coming, but it is something everyone needs to be aware of.

FAILURE is your greatest friend! Students hate to fail. Doctors hate it even more. We are told over and over that in order to get accepted into medical school we must get that 4.0 GPA and never make a mistake. Teachers get upset when we fail. Parents sometimes even yell at their children when they fail. Not just in school, but in everything in life. And that is the biggest mistake anyone can ever make.

We need to fail. We must fail. WHY? Because failure is how we learn. We learned to walk by falling down. We learned to speak by talking goobly-gock. We learned to hit a tennis ball by missing.

Hopefully you know the old story of Thomas Edison who said that his first 10,000 tries at inventing the light bulb (which ended in failures) were not failure, just ways to not invent the light bulb. He learned from his mistakes. So must we.

Everything I know comes from 3 sources – (1) reading of books, (2) other people I have met, and (3) my mistakes. It is my belief that the most important of the three is the last, because it is what I learned from my mistakes that has given me what little wisdom I possess. I bet it's the same with you.

Here's a quiz for you: Name 3 things you learned in high school that are important to you now. Not much comes to mind from your classes does it, but a lot most likely comes from some of the mistakes you made way back when.

Your child is headed for a career as a doctor. People go to doctors with their problems. Every so often I will be sitting with a patient and thinking to myself, *"Wow, that's a heck of a problem, and you're coming to me to solve it!"* *"Man, you do have problems!"*

Why am I so special to be solving their problems? All I did was get that 4.0 GPA and go to medical school. That does not make me wise. What makes me wise is what I learned along the way from my experiences, my study, but most importantly from my mistakes.

No matter where your child may be in his or her development, one of the greatest skills you can teach is that of learning from mistakes. Condemnation and pointing a finger goes nowhere.

Criticism and scolding most often do not help. Treating your child with respect and dignity is what works. No one fails on purpose. Failure can and should be used as a tool for improvement and the learning of that skill starts at home, with you – the parent. (Gee, I sound wise, but I'm not sure if that's wisdom or not.)

Your child's greatest asset is you and what you have taught. If your child can learn from failure, you have done well.

If you child says, *"Ah, that's why I screwed up,"* then you have done well. If your child has the courage to try new things, climb higher, strive for more and reach a destiny that is only a dream, then you have done well. You have done well when your child says to you,

"Dad, I think I might want to be a doctor" or also this: *"Dad, I don't think I really want to be a doctor."* Then you will know that you have done well.

SECTION III
DEVELOPING YOUR PERSONAL
PREMED TEAM

Why Do You Even Need a PreMed Team?

This third and final section may contain the most important information I can provide to parents as they consider a career of medicine for their child. Medicine is a Team Sport! PreMed as we know it today is a Solo Endeavor.

I cannot think of anything more important to anyone, other than their personal health and their family, than that of choosing a career. Especially a career that costs hundreds of thousands of dollars, years and years to get into, and that lasts upwards of fifty years.

Ronald Kapp, MD, PhD

Just as I struggled many years ago in making this decision, today's PreMed faces a similar and yet even more demanding of a choice. Still we leave it to them and them alone.

This may be the greatest dereliction of duty that I can imagine. What team could win a National Championship without their coaching and support staff? How could any golfer, tennis pro, race car driver, jockey, or any other great athlete attain winning status without their coaches and support staff?

PreMed is as grueling, or more so, than many of those and yet we allow your 18, 19, or 20 year old child to go off to college and "see what happens." Hope, as they say, is not a good strategy for success.

There is no PreMed Team on campus. Many schools provide access to the "premedical club" and nearly all campuses provide free access to the "premedical advisory staff." Fun if you are looking for fun; nearly worthless if your goal is winning the PreMed Tournament. It's the most competitive, demanding and difficult major on campus, your classmates are your direct competition. So let's all get together and party!

Now I love parties as much as anyone, but when it comes to my wellbeing and financial future, then I am all business. PreMed is business. Serious business if you ask me. Parties are fine and there's a time for that too (hey, I was at Woodstock – the biggest party ever, although I may be the only living survivor who did not use drugs that weekend). But when it comes to career and future, seriousness and winning are what count.

Winning in the PreMed World is all about having others think you are one of the best. One of the smartest, most passionate and dedicated students on campus. You are a leader and a follower at the same time. You are persistent, faithful and honest. You are a Renaissance persona of the 21st century and PreMed is what you live for. You are a test-taking-machine and you love it. And your GPA and MCAT scores prove all that and more. And lastly, you have traveled to the moon and back, twice, just for fun.

I think you get the point. It's tough and any help at all is going to pay big dividends in helping your child get that coveted acceptance letter into medical school.

It is my opinion that the best way to accomplish that goal is via a PreMed Team. A group of people is always stronger with many minds dedicated to accomplishing that one goal. Your child will still be the final arbiter and the one doing all the hard work, but the team will be there for support, guidance and direction when needed.

Having the personal support of dedicated and trusted team members goes a long way in taking some of the pressure off in trying to figure out this PreMed process and what makes for the best application. In other words, doing it alone is lowering your child's chances of success.

Many do it alone; in fact, I have seen many succeed even in spite of the condemnation of parents and friends. But overall, a team is always going to win more often that a solo competitor. How many CEOs of big corporations attained that position without the support of several insiders, personal mentors, and a strong backing by many on the Board of Directors? Not to mention the fact that your child is just starting out on that difficult career path and all we seem to be doing on most campuses is throwing them into a shark infested tank and watching to see who will sink and who will swim.

I am a firm believer that the strong will survive, they will swim, but let's at least give your child a fighting chance to prove his mettle.

That is where the concept of a PreMed Team comes in. Nobody has the ability to predict the future. Neither you, nor I, nor your children know with certainty what is going to happen tomorrow. Therefore, we cannot predict with certainty that a medical school acceptance letter is guaranteed.

However, steps and decisions can be taken that will start the ball moving in that direction and that will hopefully lead to that conclusion.

That's where the power of the team concept comes into play. The experience and years of wisdom learned from a lifetime of living can be put to good use in helping your child make the necessary decisions needed in today's competitive world. Your child, as smart as he or she might be, simply does not have the years of experience that many older people have.

Years of experience in making decisions and watching the various outcomes that arise from those decisions. That's beneficial and powerful in the PreMed Race to Acceptance and beyond. If done properly, building a personal PreMed Team can be extremely empowering to your child.

How to Start Building Your Personal PreMed Team

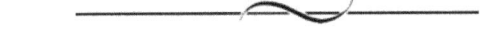

Most undergraduate students on campus have never thought about the concept of a PreMed Team. Since it doesn't exist on campus, nobody is talking about it, and the premedical advisor knows little to nothing about it, your child is clueless on the value of this team concept. In fact, I would suggest that you not even publicize the knowledge that your child is a member of an elite PreMed Team – it's your secret weapon, so to speak, on winning this race.

Therefore, the very first thing you must do is talk to your child.

Discuss the concept and "ask" him or her if this is something that seems worthwhile. You will get some resistance here because not only is this something new that nobody else is doing, but it also seems a bit intimidating and perhaps even overwhelming.

Who has time for a team? Why do I have to rely on others? What do they know that I don't know? How can they know what I want out of my life? Have they been to medical school? Are they doctors? These are just a few of the typical responses you will get from your child. It goes on and on.

Just know that if you start hearing those types of responses, then your child needs a team far more than you ever thought!

Here's why: You child is already part of a team. You and your child have been a team for the past several decades. You have been looking out for his or her welfare for many years. Yes, perhaps there were times of trouble, times of despair, times of conflict and maybe even times of estrangement, but through it all – you were there! I know it sounds corny, but it's true.

The resistance you meet is more likely a reflection of his or her wanting to be independent and free. Especially, and finally, free of those darn parents! But that's just a reflection of life, growing up and hormones.

Again, there's an old joke of one young adult talking to another: "Boy, when I was 16, it was amazing how stupid my parents were. But now that I'm 21, it's even more amazing how much they learned this past 5 years."

So your first action is to talk to your child. You need buy-in. Without that, you will go nowhere. If your child is not on-board, your chances of a successful team are basically nil. Zero. Zilch. Nada.

You can talk about your familial team. You can talk about the fact that medicine is a team sport. You can talk about how much improved chances of acceptance will be via a team effort. You can talk about team experiences, wisdom and help in making decisions. And you can talk yourself blue because if your child has no interest, then there is no interest.

But don't give up. Since you and your child are already a team, you are simply having a small team dispute about what other things might be needed.

This is an excellent learning opportunity for your child. Leave him alone. Don't bug her. Don't nag. Don't yell. Don't demand. Simply have your heart-to-heart discussion and then let it be. Let it germinate.

Allow this concept of a PreMed Team to grow and develop on its own. Remember: it's not on campus, so it is out of the ordinary.

SECTION III - How to Start Building Your Personal PreMed Team

Whatever happens, always remember: Your child is always the Team Captain. Always! It's his, or her, career, life and final decision. You are only a supporting team member. You can still support with your emotions, encouragement, and maybe even a little money on the side.

This is a fantastic learning opportunity for everyone – your child will (hopefully) eventually become a doctor and be the leader of that medical team. He/she will have to learn how to listen to, and take advice from nurses (banish the thought), administrators (golly, not that), insurance carriers (heavens no), and most important of all – minimum-wage-paid secretarial staff (is there no justice in this world) that control a doctor's life.

If your child is so recalcitrant now in not wanting to form a PreMed Team to help get accepted into medical school, I shudder to think how miserable and unhappy he, and she, will be whence they are real doctors!

On the other hand, hopefully your child will seriously consider the PreMed Team concept and come to the logical conclusion that more minds are better than one. Come to the conclusion that experiences and wisdom can be useful. Come to the conclusion that greatness and success nearly always rest on the shoulders of those who went before us.

Your child should see himself as that great athlete who wins a Gold Medal at the Olympics, but knows deep in his heart that is was a team effort all along. Your child is the star. Your child will be doing the heavy lifting.

Your child will become that test-taking-machine of a maniac studying to become a doctor, but you and your other team members will be there right behind him. Basking in the glory that comes with your offspring successfully getting accepted into medical school.

Ronald Kapp, MD, PhD

But you and your child rarely can do it alone. You need more team members. So who do you add and how do you go about adding more team members, your coaching staff so to speak?

Who and How to Add Team Members

Once again, the first thing you must remember is that your child is Always the Team Captain; you are only a supporting staff member. You can suggest, but you cannot demand. You can advise, but you cannot dictate. You can recommend, but you cannot rule. To do otherwise is to do a great disservice to the developing leadership potential of your child.

That's another reason why so many of today's physicians hate their career, they never learned how to be true leaders. They are instead dictators. They dictate this, they dictate that. Gee, I wonder where they learned that behavior, Mom, Dad?

True Leaders lead by example, others follow them eagerly, gladly and freely. True Leaders listen to others, they take under consideration what others tell them and then they make a decision. That is what every doctor does every day, day in and day out. Only some are dictators and big surprise here, they hate their jobs.

The first additional team member is a no-brainer. That will be the campus premedical advisor. What, heresy you say. I thought they knew nothing! No, I did not say that. I said they know nothing about clinical medicine and being a practicing doctor. But they know everything about the PreMed Application Process, the course requirements, how to get letters of recommendation, when and how to sign up for the MCAT, how to submit those multiple med school applications, etc. They know all the day-to-day operational requirements needed to successfully navigate the application process.

That person, or campus committee, must be actively recruited as a team member. I would suggest, and this is a KEY CONCEPT – that you not even tell that person he or she is a team member! They will, and must, so decline! Think about it – how could that person be a team member of your team, and not a team member of every other student on campus?

Their job is to provide a service to all students, equally, non-discriminatorily, and unbiased to every student who enters the premedical office. If that person becomes an official team member of your PreMed Team, they get fired from the university! Do you understand that? That person is, however, a vitally important behind-the-scene team member, even if not consciously aware of so being or not.

The campus advisor is super important. Your child needs to meet and greet that person ASAP. Today is okay, yesterday would have been better. A long term relationship is always better than *"Hi, I'm a senior with a 3.7 GPA and I want to go to medical school."* Surprisingly, that's how it happens more often than not. But then remember that more than 50% of our practicing doctors really hate their choice of a career.

Your campus advisor does know a lot about the application process and also a lot about students wanting to become doctors. They should know tons of things after a few years of seeing hundreds, if not thousands, of applicants enter the meat-grinder of becoming-a-doctor.

I call it a meat-grinder because that is how it often seems to students as they progress farther and farther down the road – they enter, but they can't get out. They already have too much invested in the process (time, effort and money) to ever back out and say – I quit. It's a meat-grinder and that is why your child's inner passion, motivation, and deep undying desires are so important. Without that passion, the meat-grinder will turn your child into hamburger meat, and not that delicious delicacy of a mushroom I talked about earlier. And the campus advisor is a stop along that journey.

After that, team member selection becomes a very individualized selection process. I leave this up to your own imagination because each student is a unique asset base which you are growing.

I might suggest that the next member could be a "trusted family friend." That person would have your child's best interests at heart, but be one step removed from familial emotions and therefore able to provide valuable insight.

Another selection might be some type of professional person, such as a doctor or lawyer. This person has been through the educational meat-grinder in some format and has a unique perspective on what it takes to accomplish what your child is trying to do.

Another selection might be a successful businessperson who understands competition and how the world works. Another good selection type might be someone from the clergy who has a more philosophical slant on how life works.

And of course don't ever forget someone who is in your own child's age and status group who you can implicitly trust. Each final student PreMed Team will be a unique blend of who you know, trust and have access to. There is no set formula for who should or should not be on a team.

How to add a team member is a rather interesting process. Obviously, these are people you already know and trust. This is your child's future you are talking about. Each member must want and be willing to help. They too must have buy-in, just as did your child. The only way to find that out is to ask. Ask and explain. Explain what you want them to be doing. Ask if they have the time and inclination. Ask if this is something they feel comfortable doing. Ask if they have the passion for doing this.

What Exactly Will the PreMed Team Members Be Doing Anyway?

That's exactly what anyone you ask will ask you. What do you want me to do? If someone doesn't ask that upfront, you may have a problem and need to reconsider if this is someone you really want on the team.

Being a team member is a super-important position to your child's career. You don't want a dictator, you don't want a know-it-all, and you don't want someone who is not interested in your child's future.

What you want is that person's knowledge, experience and wisdom. You want someone both you and your child trust and can easily work with. Someone you both respect. Someone who wants to help. And guess what – it's easily than you think.

Firstly, they will be acting in your child's best interest. That is rule number one. They must have an interest in wanting your child to succeed. They must be open-minded and willing to listen to your child.

Remember your child remains the Team Captain. Team members work for him or her. Some team members will do it for free, others must be paid.

Secondly, they must make some time to be available to meet with your child. This can be in person, or even digitally via the internet. It does not have to be much time, but it has to be quality time. Quality trumps quantity.

Thirdly, they must understand what your child is trying to accomplish. The true goal is two-fold: Getting accepted into medical school is part 1, and becoming a successful, happy practicing physician is part 2. You can easily have the first, without the second. Your goal is to have both.

Fourthly, they must have wisdom. Fortunately, everyone has wisdom – it is not something in short supply. They do not have to know anything about medicine or medical school or even like doctors that much. But they have to know a little about life itself. That is wisdom.

And lastly, they must be honest and truthful with you. Platitudes, compliments and being a yes-sir-type-of-person does you no good long term. Sweet compliments might feel good today, but this is an epic journey of gargantuan importance and you want the truth – You Can Handle the Truth!

The truth is that getting an acceptance into medical school is really not that difficult. Getting through medical school is even easier. Practicing medicine is where the rubber hits the road.

Today's doctor shortage is only going to worsen, but even worse is the fact that over 50% of practicing physicians would not do it over again if given the chance. Your goal, and that of your child, is to not be in that group.

Your team members should be selected to see that that does not happen. They should want what is best for your son or daughter – sometimes doctoring is a destiny, sometimes not. Glamour and glitz should not drive destiny, a personal calling should.

A personal calling to be a wise healer that alleviates the suffering of others is a destiny worth years of effort. It is a challenge like no other.

SECTION III - What the PreMed Team Members Be Doing

It is a mountain of education to be climbed, with a view seen by a few privileged students who have made their calling a dream of reality. People you ask to join your team can share in that dream and make it reality.

Ronald Kapp, MD, PhD

Why Do I Coach PreMed Students?

I believe the most influential movie of my life was "The Man Who Planted Trees." If you have not seen the movie, the moral is this: The story of one shepherd's long and successful singlehanded effort to re-forest a desolate valley.

Deep personal reflection has revealed to me that the most pivotal point in my destiny was that of "getting accepted into medical school." That seed has grown into my tree-planting-mission today of helping others make a similar pivotal decision for themselves – getting the right student into the right profession.

By doing that, I will begin the process of solving our health care crisis, one doctor at a time.

This guide is an introduction to what I teach PreMed students in my *Advanced PreMed Life Support* course. Twenty years of PreMed research and a lifetime of learning how to practice medicine have been dedicated to the development of this course. It is a course like no other and is not available from anyone else. It is personal, interactive and will change your child's life.

Ronald Kapp, MD, PhD

ABOUT THE AUTHOR

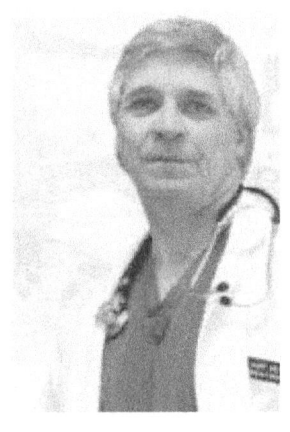

Dr. Kapp is a practicing physician with more than 85,000 hours of emergency room experience. He is a national advisor, mentor and coach who created the Advanced PreMed Life Support Course for undergraduate students. He also regularly provides coaching to medical students, residents-in-training and International Medical Graduates (IMG's). He will be your personal mentor and coach in helping you get accepted into medical school.

KAPPMD, INC. is a boutique advisory practice focused on increasing the performance of undergraduate premedical students, medical students and physicians-in-training. Founded by practicing physician Ronald Kapp, MD, PhD in 2002, this pragmatic approach to preparing tomorrow's physician focuses on practical, actionable skills needed to compete in today's complex world of medicine.

Ronald Kapp, MD, PhD

Through his own direct experience as a physician and advisor, and with over two decades of extensive research, Dr. Kapp is passionately convinced that personal actions and behaviors can be modeled to enhance the performance of our future doctors. A sought-after and compelling speaker and advisor, he delivers a message of passion and dedication to the profession so that individuals may benefit from his experience.

KAPPMD, INC. offers individual advisory services and custom consulting to students dedicated to the medical profession. Dr. Kapp has personally developed his unique course – Advanced PreMed Life Support (APLS) as the only course available specifically dedicated to getting undergraduate students accepted into medical school and prepared for a successful and rewarding career as a physician.

CONTACT

For more information on the Advanced Premed Life Support Program contact Dr. Kapp at: drkapp@kappmd.com

Or visit: www.kappmd.com

Ronald Kapp, MD, PhD

Other Books by Dr. Ron Kapp

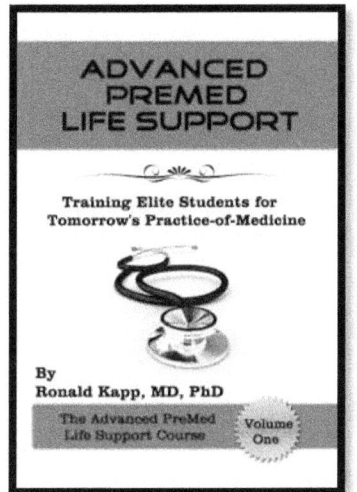

Advanced PreMed Life Support

Training Elite Students for Tomorrow's Practice-of-Medicine

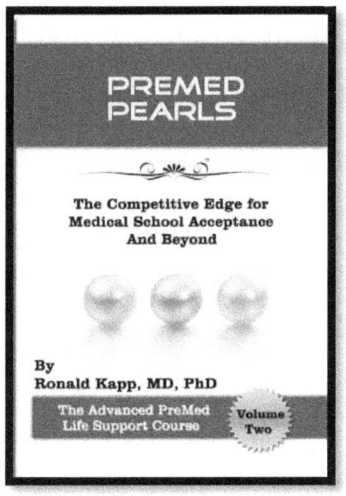

PreMed Pearls

For the elite premedical student. Learn about the medical profession from practicing physicians – wisdom, motivation, and inspiration.

Ronald Kapp, MD, PhD

Index

www.ingramcontent.com/pod-product-compliance
Lightning Source LLC
Chambersburg PA
CBHW070107210526
45170CB00013B/780